HOW TO PLAY:

STEP 1:
GATHER UP ALL YOUR FRIENDS AND ALCOHOL.

STEP 2:
ON EACH PAGE YOU WILL HAVE 3 QUESTIONS. ASK ONE FRIEND AT A TIME TO PICK A NUMBER BETWEEN 1-3.

STEP 3:
THE FRIEND CAN RATHER ANSWER THE QUESTION OR TAKE A DRINK/SHOT.

Loading ...

LETS START WITH A FEW EASY ONES

TRUTH OR DRINK...

1. HAVE YOU EVER HAD SEX IN A CAR?

2. HAVE YOU EVER BEEN ATTRACTED TO THE SAME SEX?

3. HAVE YOU EVER CHEATED/WANTED TO CHEAT?

4.

TRUTH OR DRINK...

1. WHEN WAS YOUR FIRST KISS?

2. HAVE YOU EVER KISSED SOMEONE IN THIS ROOM?

3. WHERE IS THE WEIRDEST PLACE YOU HAVE MADE OUT?

TRUTH OR DRINK...

1. WHEN WAS THE LAST TIME YOU HAD SEX?

2. HAVE YOU EVER HAD SEX WITH ANYONE IN THIS ROOM?

3. WHO DO YOU REGRET HAVING SEX WITH?

TRUTH OR DRINK...

1. HAVE YOU FARTED IN THE LAST HOUR?

2. HAVE YOU EVER FARTED DURING SEX?

3. WHEN ALONE, DO YOU SMELL YOUR OWN FARTS AND ENJOY IT?

TRUTH OR DRINK...

1. WHEN DID YOU LAST HAVE A POO?

2. HOW SMELLY WAS YOUR LAST POO?

3. DESCRIBE IN DETAIL THE WORST POO YOU'VE EVER HAD.

TRUTH OR DRINK...

1. NAME 1 CELEBRITY YOU WOULD SLEEP WITH.

2. NAME 3 CELEBRITIES YOU WOULD SLEEP WITH.

3. NAME 5 CELEBRITIES YOU WOULD SLEEP WITH.

TRUTH OR DRINK...

1. WHAT DO YOU REALLY THINK ABOUT THE PERSON ASKING THIS QUESTION?

2. WHAT DO YOU REALLY THINK ABOUT THE PERSON ON YOUR LEFT?

3. WHAT DO YOU REALLY THINK ABOUT THE PERSON ON YOUR RIGHT?

TRUTH OR DRINK...

1. HOW MUCH PORN DO YOU WATCH IN A WEEK?

2. WHAT IS THE WEIRDEST PORN YOU GENRE YOU WATCH?

3. WHEN WAS THE LAST TIME YOU WATCHED PORN?

TRUTH OR DRINK...

1. PUT EVERYONE IN ORDER OF WHO YOU WOULD SLEEP WITH.

2. PUT EVERYONE IN ORDER OF WHO YOU WOULD UNFRIEND.

3. PUT EVERYONE IN ORDER OF WHO YOU WOULD KISS.

TRUTH OR DRINK...

1. WHAT SONG GETS YOU IN THE MOOD?

2. WHAT MOVIE GETS YOU IN THE MOOD?

3. WHAT IS IT SOMEONE CAN DO TO GET YOU IN THE MOOD?

TRUTH OR DRINK...

1. HAVE YOU EVER HAD SEX WITH SOMEONE OF THE SAME SEX?

2. HAVE YOU EVER HAD AN ORGY?

3. HAVE YOU EVER HAD A THREESOME?

TRUTH OR DRINK...

1. HAVE YOU EVER BEEN SICK AND THEN MADE OUT WITH SOMEONE?

2. HAVE YOU EVER MADE OUT WITH SOMEONE WHO CLEARLY JUST WAS SICK?

3. WHAT'S YOUR WORST VOMIT STORY?

TRUTH OR DRINK...

1. HAVE YOU EVER HAD SEX WITH SOMEONE IN THIS ROOM?

2. HAVE YOU EVER HAD SEX WITH YOUR FRIENDS EX?

3. HAVE YOU EVER HAD SEX WITH SOMEONE YOUR FRIEND HAD A CRUSH ON?

TRUTH OR DRINK...

1. WHAT IS THE KINKIEST THING YOU HAVE DONE?

2. WHAT IS YOUR WEIRD FETISH?

3. HAS ANYONE YOU HAVE BEEN WITH HAD A WEIRD FETISH?

TRUTH OR DRINK...

1. NAME 1 FRIEND YOU WOULD SLEEP WITH.

2. NAME 3 FRIENDS YOU WOULD SLEEP WITH.

3. NAME 5 FRIENDS YOU WOULD SLEEP WITH.

TRUTH OR DRINK...

1. WHAT IS YOUR LEAST FAVOURITE SEX POSITION?

2. WHAT IS YOUR FAVOURITE SEX POSITION?

3. WHAT SEX POSTION DO YOU WANT TO TRY?

TRUTH OR DRINK...

1. DESCRIBE YOUR LAST HEARTBREAK.

2. ARE YOU STILL IN LOVE WITH AN EX?

3. DO YOU STILL THINK ABOUT SEX WITH AN EX?

TRUTH OR DRINK...

1. DO/DID YOU HAVE A PET NAME?

2. DO YOU HAVE PET NAMES FOR CURRENT/EX PARTNERS?

3. WHAT IS THE WEIRDEST PET NAME YOU'VE BEEN CALLED?

TRUTH OR DRINK...

1. HAVE YOU EVER SEEN A FRIENDS NUDES?

2. HAVE A FRIEND EVER SEEN YOUR NUDES?

3. HAVE YOU EVER SENT A NUDE TO THE WRONG PERSON?

TRUTH OR DRINK...

1. SAY HOW MUCH IT WOULD COST FOR YOU TO SLEEP WITH EACH PERSON.

2. WOULD YOU EVER HAVE SEX FOR MONEY?

3. WOULD YOU EVER DO PORN?

24.

LETS REALLY GET TO KNOW YOUR FRIENDS

25.

TRUTH OR DRINK...

1. WHEN WAS THE LAST TIME YOU MASTERBATED?

2. WHAT WAS THE LAST THING YOU MASTERBATED OVER?

3. WHAT WAS THE WEIRDEST THING YOU HAVE EVER MASTERBATED OVER?

TRUTH OR DRINK...

1. WHEN DID YOU LOSE YOUR VIRGINITY?

2. HOW MANY PEOPLE HAVE YOU SLEPT WITH?

3. DESCRIBE IN DETAIL THE LAST TIME YOU HAD SEX.

TRUTH OR DRINK...

1. HAVE YOU EVER BEEN CAUGHT IN THE ACT?

2. HAVE YOU EVER WALKED IN ON SOMEONE HAVING SEX?

3. HAVE YOU EVER HEARD ANYONE IN THE ROOM HAVE SEX?

TRUTH OR DRINK...

1. HAVE YOU EVER HAD SEX OUTSIDE?

2. DO YOU WANT TO HAVE SEX OUTSIDE?

3. DO YOU/WOULD YOU HAVE SEX WHILE PEOPLE WATCH?

TRUTH OR DRINK...

1. HAVE YOU EVER PAID FOR SEX?

2. WOULD YOU EVER PAY FOR SEX?

3. WHAT SEXUAL THINGS WOULD YOU DO FOR MONEY?

TRUTH OR DRINK...

1. TELL THE PERSON ON YOUR LEFT THE FILTHIEST THING YOU CAN SEE THEM DOING.

2. TELL THE PERSON ON YOUR RIGHT THE FILTHIEST THING YOU CAN SEE THEM DOING.

3. TELL EVERYONE IN THE ROOM WHAT THE FILTHIEST THING YOU CAN SEE THEM DOING.

TRUTH OR DRINK...

1. DESCRIBE WHAT IS WAS LIKE THE FIRST TIME SOMEONE GAVE YOU ORAL.

2. DESCRIBE WHAT IT WAS LIKE THE LAST TIME SOMEONE GAVE YOU ORAL.

3. DESCRIBE WHAT IT WAS LIKE THE WORST TIME SOMEONE GAVE YOU ORAL.

TRUTH OR DRINK...

1. HAVE YOU EVER THOUGHT ABOUT SEX AT WORK?

2. HAVE YOU EVER HAD SEX AT WORK?

3. HAVE YOU EVER MASTERBATED AT WORK?

TRUTH OR DRINK...

1. TELL EVERYONE WHAT WAS THE REASON WHY YOU LAST CRIED.

2. TELL EVERYONE WHAT WAS THE REASON WHY YOU WAS LAST SAD.

3. TELL EVERYONE WHAT WAS THE REASON WHY YOU WAS LAST HORNY.

TRUTH OR DRINK...

1. WHO DO YOU LOVE?

2. WHO IS YOUR SECRET CRUSH?

3. WHO DO YOU REALLY WANT TO HAVE SEX WITH?

TRUTH OR DRINK...

1. WHER ON THE BODY DO YOU LIKE TO BE KISSED?

2. WHERE ON THE BODY DO YOU NOT LIKE TO BE KISSED?

3. DO YOU HAVE A FOOT FETISH?

TRUTH OR DRINK...

1. HAVE YOU EVER BEEN CATFISHED?

2. HAVE YOU EVER CATFISHED ANYONE?

3. DO YOU KNOW SOMEONE WHO HAS SECRETLY CATFISHED SOMEONE?

TRUTH OR DRINK...

1. DO YOU LIKE TO BE TIED UP?

2. DO YOU LIKE TO USE HANDCUFFS?

3. DO YOU LIKE TO USE WHIPS?

TRUTH OR DRINK...

1. DESCRIBE YOUR FUNNIEST CUM STORY.

2. DESCRIBE YOUR MOST AWKWARD CUM STORY.

3. DESCRIBE THE LAST TIME YOU FAKED IT.

TRUTH OR DRINK...

1. HAVE YOU EVER HAD A CRUSH ON A TEACHER?

2. HAVE YOU EVER HAD A CRUSH ON A COUSIN?

3. HAVE YOU EVER HAD A CRUSH ON ONE OF YOUR FRIENDS FAMILY MEMBER?

TRUTH OR DRINK...

1. WOULD YOU GO BACK TO AN EX?

2. WOULD YOU HAVE SEX WITH YOUR BEST FRIENDS EX?

3. WOULD YOU HAVE SEX WITH ONE OF YOUR FRIENDS CURRENT PARTNER?

TRUTH OR DRINK...

1. WHAT WAS THE LAST SEXUAL CONVERSATION ABOUT?

2. WHO WAS THE LAST PERSON YOU HAD A SEXUAL CONVERSATION WITH.- BEFORE THIS GAME.

3. DO YOU DO SEXTING?

TRUTH OR DRINK...

1. ASK THE PERSON ON YOUR LEFT IF THEY WOULD HAVE SEX WITH YOU.- IF REFUSE, BOTH DRINK,

2. ASK THE PERSON ASKING THIS QUESTION IF THEY WOULD HAVE SEX WITH YOU.- IF REFUSE, BOTH DRINK

3. ASK THE PERSON ON YOUR RIGHT IF THEY WOULD HAVE SEX WITH YOU.- IF REFUSE, BOTH DRINK.

TRUTH OR DRINK...

1. HOW MANY PEOPLE HAVE SEEN YOU NAKED IN THIS ROOM?

2. HOW MANY PEOPLE HAVE YOU SEEN NAKED IN THIS ROOM?

3. HOW MANY PEOPLE DO YOU WANT TO SEE NAKED IN THIS ROOM?

TRUTH OR DRINK...

1. DESCRIBE IN DETAIL THE LAST NUDE YOU TOOK.

2. HAVE YOU EVER TAKEN A NUDE?

3. WHO WAS THE LAST PERSON YOU SENT A NUDE TOO?

LETS

GETS

PERSONAL

TRUTH OR DRINK...

1. SAY WHAT THE PERSON ON YOUR LEFT NEEDS TO DO TO IMPROVE THEIR LIFE.

2. SAY WHAT THE PERSON WHO IS ASKING THIS QUESTION NEEDS TO DO TO IMPROVE THEIR LIFE.

3. SAY WHAT THE PERSON ON YOUR RIGHT NEEDS TO DO TO IMPROVE THEIR LIFE.

TRUTH OR DRINK...

1. ASK EVERYONE IF THEY HAVE EVER THOUGHT ABOUT YOU NAKED. - IF THEY REFUSE, DRINK.

2. TELL THE PERSON IN THE ROOM THAT YOU HAVE THOUGHT ABOUT NAKED.

3. HAVE YOU EVER HAD A SEX DREAM ABOUT ANYONE IN THE ROOM?

TRUTH OR DRINK...

1. TELL THE PERSON ON YOUR RIGHT WHAT YOU DON'T LIKE ABOUT THEM.

2. TELL THE PERSON ON YOUR LEFT WHAT YOU DON'T LIKE ABOUT THEM.

3. TELL THE PERSON ASKING THE QUESTIONS WHAT YOU DON'T LIKE ABOUT THEM.

TRUTH OR DRINK...

1. DO YOU OWN A SEX TOY?

2. HAVE YOU EVER USED A SEX TOY DURING SEX?

3. ARE YOU INTO BDSM?

TRUTH OR DRINK...

1. DESCRIBE IN DETAIL YOUR PRIVATE PARTS.

2. DESCRIBE IN DETAIL THE PRIVATE PARTS OF THE LAST PERSON YOU HAVE SEX WITH.

3. DO YOU SHAVE YOUR PRIVATE PARTS?

TRUTH OR DRINK...

1. ASK THE PERSON ON YOUR RIGHT WHAT THEY DON'T LIKE ABOUT YOU.- IF REFUSE, BOTH DRINK.

2. ASK THE PERSON ON YOUR LEFT WHAT THEY DONT LIKE ABOUT YOU.- IF REFUSE, BOTH DRINK.

3. WHAT DON'T YOU LIKE ABOUT YOURSELF?

TRUTH OR DRINK...

1. DO YOU LIKE ANAL?

2. DO YOU GIVE ORAL?

3. DO YOU DO 69?

TRUTH OR DRINK...

1. DESCRIBE THE BEST SEXUAL FANTASY YOU HAVE DONE.

2. DESCRIBE THE WORST SEXUAL FANTASY YOU HAVE DONE.

3. DESCRIBE THE SEXUAL FANTASY YOU WANT TO TRY.

TRUTH OR DRINK...

1. WHAT IS THE MOST TIMES YOU'VE HAD SEX IN ONE DAY?

2. WHAT IS THE MOST TIMES YOU'VE MASTERBATED IN ONE DAY?

3. WHAT'S THE MOST TIMES YOU'VE CUM IN ONE SEXUAL INTERCOURSE?

TRUTH OR DRINK...

1. ASK THE PERSON ON THE LEFT WHAT THEY LOVE ABOUT YOU.- DRINK TO IT.

2. ASK THE PERSON WHO IS ASKING THIS QUESTION WHAT THEY LOVE ABOUT YOU.- DRINK TO IT.

3. ASK THE PERSON ON THE RIGHT WHAT THEY LOVE ABOUT YOU.- DRINK TO IT.

TRUTH OR DRINK...

1. TELL THE PERSON ON YOUR RIGHT WHAT THE MOST SEXUAL THING YOU WOULD DO WITH THEM IS.

2. TELL THE PERSON ON YOUR LEFT WHAT THE MOST SEXUAL THING YOU WOULD DO WITH THEM IS.

3. TELL THE PERSON ASKING THIS QUESTION WHAT IS THE MOST SEXUAL THING YOU WOULD DO WITH THEM IS.

TRUTH OR DRINK...

1. TELL EACH PERSON IN THE ROOM WHAT THEIR BEST FEATURE IS.

2. TELL EACH PERSON IN THE ROOM WHAT YOU THINK THEIR PRIVATE PARTS LOOK LIKE.

3. TELL EACH PERSON IN THE ROOM WHAT SEX WOULD BE LIKE WITH THEM.

TRUTH OR DRINK...

1. TELL EVERYONE A SECRET HOOK UP THAT NO ONE KNOWS ABOUT.

2. TELL EVERYONE A SECRET DIRTY TEXT MESSAGE NO ONE KNOWS ABOUT

3. TELL EVERYONE A SECRET YOU KEEPING FOR A FRIEND.

TRUTH OR DRINK...

1. HAVE YOU EVER STOLEN ANYTHING FROM SOMEONE IN THIS ROOM?

2. HAVE YOU EVER STOLEN FROM YOUR PARENTS?

3. HAVE YOU EVER STOLEN ANYTHING FROM A FRIEND THATS NOT HERE?

TRUTH OR DRINK...

1. HOW OFTEN DO YOU SHAVE YOUR PRIVATES?

2. DO YOU LIKE THE OTHER PERSON TO BE SHAVEN?

3. ARE YOUR PRIVATES SHAVED RIGHT NOW?

TRUTH OR DRINK...

1. WHAT IS THE WEIRDEST THING YOU'VE PUT IN SOMEONES BODY?

2. WHAT IS THE WEIRDEST THING YOU'VE PUT IN YOUR BODY?

3. WHAT IS ONE THING YOU WANT TO TRY PUTTING IN YOUR BODY?

TRUTH OR DRINK...

1. HAVE YOU EVER HAD A STD?

2. HAVE YOU EVER GONE TO THE HOSPITAL FOR A SEXUAL REASON?

3. HAVE YOU EVER STRUGGLED TO PERSFORM? OR THE OTHER PERSON COULDN'T PERFORM?

TRUTH OR DRINK...

1. WHAT IS THE SIZE OF YOUR BREASTS/PENIS?

2. WHAT WAS THE SIZE OF THE BREASTS/PENIS OF THE PERSON YOU LAST HAD SEX WITH?

3. DO YOU WISH YOUR BREASTS/PENIS WAS BIGGER?

TRUTH OR DRINK...

1. LET THE PERSON ON THE LEFT ASK YOU A SEXUAL QUESTION THEY'VE ALWAYS WANTED TO KNOW.

2. LET THE PERSON ON THE RIGHT ASK YOU A SEXUAL QUESTION THEY'VE ALWAYS WANTED TO KNOW.

3. LET THE PERSON ASKING THIS QUESTION ASK YOU A SEXUAL QUESTION THEY'VE ALWAYS WANTED TO KNOW.

TRUTH OR DRINK...

1. DESCRIBE IN DETAIL THE BEST SEX YOU'VE EVER HAD.

2. DESCRIBE IN DETAIL THE WORST SEX YOU'VE EVER HAD.

3. DESCRIBE IN DETAIL THE LAST TIME YOU HAD SEX.

NOW THAT WE
ARE ON PAGE 69,

SHALL WE DO
A FEW DARES?

TRUTH OR DRINK...

1. WITH CLOTHES ON, THIS ISN'T AN ORGY, CHOOSE SOMEONE TO GET INTO THE 69 POSITION WITH.

2. CHOOSE SOMEONE TO GET INTO YOUR FAVOURITE SEX POSITION.

3. CHOOSE SOMEONE AND GET INTO THEIR FAVOURITE SEX POSTION.

TRUTH OR DRINK...

1. ALLOW THE PERSON ON THE LEFT GO THROUGH YOUR TEXTS ON YOUR PHONE.

2. ALLOW THE PERSON ON YOUR RIGHT GO THROUGH YOUR PICTURES ON YOUR PHONE.

3. ALLOW THE PERSON ASKING THE QUESTION GO THROUGH YOUR PHONE.

TRUTH OR DRINK...

1. KISS THE PERSON ON YOUR LEFT.

2. KISS THE PERSON READING THE QUESTION.

3. KISS THE PERSON ON YOUR RIGHT.

TRUTH OR DRINK...

1. GIVE SOMEONE A SEXY DANCE.

2. DO YOUR BEST TWERKING. SHAKE THAT BUTT.

3. CHOOSE SOMEONE TO GIVE YOU A SEXY DANCE. - THEY CAN DRINK TO GET OUT OF IT.

TRUTH OR DRINK...

1. DO YOUR BEST CHAT-UP LINE TO THE PERSON ON YOUR LEFT.

2. DO YOUR BEST CHAT-UP LINE TO THE PERSON ON YOUR RIGHT.

3. DO YOUR BEST CHAT-UP LINE TO THE PERSON YOU FIND MOST ATTRACTIVE.

TRUTH OR DRINK...

1. CALL YOUR EX TO TELL THEM YOU WANT TO GET BACK TOGETHER.

2. TEXT YOUR EX TO TELL THEM YOU WANT TO GET BACK TOGETHER.

3. ALLOW THE PERSON READING THE QUESTION TEXT YOUR EX.

TRUTH OR DRINK...

1. DO YOUR BEST ORGASM NOISE.

2. MAKE THE SOUNDS OF THE LAST PERSON YOU HAD SEX WITH.

3. CHOOSE SOMEONE TO DO THEIR ORGASM NOISE. - THEY CAN DRINK TO GET OUT OF IT.

TRUTH OR DRINK...

1. ALLOW THE PERSON ON YOUR RIGHT TEXT WHOEVER THEY WANT ON YOUR PHONE.

2. ALLOW THE PERSON ON YOUR LEFT TEXT WHOEVER THEY WANT ON YOUR PHONE.

3. ALLOW THE PERSON ASKING THE QUESTION TEXT WHOEVER THEY WANT ON YOUR PHONE.

TRUTH OR DRINK...

1. LOOK AT THE PERSON ASKING THE QUESTION IN THE EYES AND TELL THEM YOU LOVE THEM.

2. LOOK AT THE PERSON ON YOUR RIGHT IN THE EYES AND TELL THEM YOU LOVE THEM.

3. LOOK AT THE PERSON ON YOUR LEFT IN THE EYES AND TELL THEM YOU LOVE THEM.

TRUTH OR DRINK...

1. KISS THE FEET OF PERSON ON YOUR LEFT. - BOTH HAVE TO DRINK IF THEY REFUSE

2. KISS THE FEET OF PERSON ON YOUR RIGHT. - BOTH HAVE TO DRINK IF THEY REFUSE.

3. ALLOW THE PERSON ASKING THE QUESTION CHOOSE THE PERSONS FEET TO KISS. - BOTH HAVE TO DRINK IF THEY REFUSE.

TRUTH OR DRINK...

1. GO OUTSIDE AND DO YOUR BEST ORGASM NOISE.

2. ALLOW THE PERSON ASKING THE QUESTION TO CHOOSE WHAT YOU HAVE TO DO OUTSIDE.

3. GO OUTSIDE AND SHOUT OUT YOUR CRUSH/PARTNERS NAME.

TRUTH OR DRINK...

1. POST ON A SOCIAL MEDIA: "I'M FEELING HORNY!"

2. POST ON A SOCIAL MEDIA: "JUST HAD SEX, WASN'T GREAT."

3. ALLOW THE PERSON ASKING QUESTION POST ANYTHING THEY WANT ON YOUR SOCIAL MEDIA.

TRUTH OR DRINK...

1. TAKE 3 SHOTS.

2. TAKE 2 SHOTS.

3. EVERYONE HAS TO TAKE A SHOT.

TRUTH OR DRINK...

1. ALLOW THE PERSON ON YOUR LEFT CHOOSE SOMETHING FOR YOU TO EAT. - NO FOOD. DRINK.

2. ALLOW THE PERSON ASKING THE QUESTION CHOOSE SOMETHING FOR YOU TO EAT. - NO FOOD. DRINK.

3. ALLOW THE PERSON ON YOUR RIGHT CHOOSE SOMETHING FOR YOU TO EAT. - NO FOOD. DRINK.

TRUTH OR DRINK...

1. PUT THE FINGER OF THE PERSON ON YOUR RIGHT IN YOUR MOUTH.

2. PUT THE FINGER OF THE PERSON ON YOUR LEFT IN YOUR MOUTH.

3. PUT THE FINGER OF THE PERSON READING THE QUESTION IN YOUR MOUTH.

TRUTH OR DRINK...

1. GO INT A PRIVATE ROOM WITH THE PERSON ON YOUR RIGHT AND DO WHATEVER YOU TWO WANT,

2. GO INTO A PRIVATE ROOM WITH THE PERSON ON YOUR LEFT AND DO WHATEVER YOU TWO WANT.

3. ALLOW THE PERSON ASKING THE QUESTION CHOOSE SOMEONE TO GO WITH INTO A PRIVATE ROOM AND DO WHAYEVER YOU WANT.

TRUTH OR DRINK...

1. ALLOW THE PERSON ON YOUR LEFT SIT ON YOUR LAP UNTIL THE NEXT ROUND IS OVER.

2. ALLOW THE PERSON ON YOUR RIGHT SIT ON YOUR LAP UNTIL THE NEXT ROUND IS OVER.

3. ALLOW THE PERSON ASKING THE QUESTION SIT ON YOUR LAP UNTIL THE NEXT ROUND IS OVER.

TRUTH OR DRINK...

1. ALLOW THE PERSON ASKING THE QUESTION GIVE YOU A HICKEY/LOVE BITE.

2. ALLOW THE PERSON ON YOUR RIGHT GIVE YOU A HICKEY/LOVE BITE.

3. ALLOW THE PERSON ON YOUR LEFT GIVE YOU A HICKEY/LOVE BITE.

TRUTH OR DRINK...

1. TRY AND DO YOUR BEST BURP INFRONT OF EVERYONE

2. TRY AND DO YOUR LOUDEST FART INFRONT OF EVERYONE.

3. ALLOW EVERYONE TO TRY AND BURP IN YOUR FACE.

TRUTH OR DRINK...

1. TEXT THE PERSON IN THE ROOM WHO YOU WOULD WANT TO HAVE SEX WITH.

2. TEXT THE PERSON IN THE ROOM WHO YOU WANT TO GO ON A DATE WITH.

3. EVERYONE HAS TO TEXT YOU IF THEY WOULD HAVE SEX WITH YOU. - WHOEVER REFUSES HAS TO DRINK.

GAME OVER

YOU ABSOLUTE LEGENDS!

THANK YOU FOR PURCHASING THIS BOOK. I HOPE YOU HAVE HAD A GREAT PARTY AND LEARNT MORE ABOUT YOUR FRIENDSHIPS. I HOPE YOU ARE ALL STILL FRIENDS, REMEMBER IT'S ALL A BIT OF FUN!

I APPRECIATE EVERY SINGLE ONE OF YOU!

Daniel R.S. Doyle

Made in the USA
Monee, IL
28 November 2025

36730025R10056